LEGAL

Limits of Liability / Disclaimer of Warranty:

The authors of this information and the accompanying materials have used their best efforts in preparing this course. The authors make no representation or warranties with respect to the accuracy, applicability, fitness, or completeness of the contents of this course. They disclaim any warranties (expressed or implied), merchantability, or fitness for any particular purpose. The authors shall in no event be held liable for any loss or other damages, including but not limited to special, incidental, consequential, or other damages.

This manual contains information protected under International Federal Copyright laws and Treaties. Any unauthorized reprint or use of this material is strictly prohibited. We actively search for copyright infringement and you will be prosecuted.

Introduction

What is the largest internal organ in your body? If you are reading this book, you already know it is the liver. The liver performs many functions in the body. Without it, you would not last very long. This book will focus on taking care of your liver. More importantly, weight loss through liver maintenance will be the goal we will try to communicate.

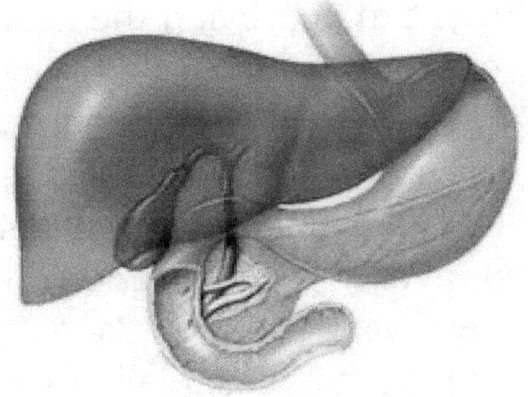

There is a direct correlation between a healthy liver and healthy weight. A toxic liver will not allow the human body to maintain a healthy, normal weighted frame. Why do men look pregnant? What does that beer belly really come from? Why do we yo-yo diet and end up putting more weight back on? A healthy liver will help you maintain a healthy weight. A poorly functioning liver will make and keep you fat. We hope the information in this book will help you make a decision to do two things in particular.

First, we want you to make a commitment to improving the health of your liver. Your life is worth it. The length of your life is tied to your liver and other vital organs. We will suggest some lifestyle changes that will help you heal your liver in a short period of time. Second, we want you to make a commitment to increasing your oxygen supply to your body. In other words; no matter what your age, you need to start exercising. You will add years to your life when you clean your liver and start an exercise program.

Read on and start your program back to
health today. We are proud of you for
making some changes in your life.
Those changes are starting here by
taking in some new information. Picture
yourself a more vibrant, energetic
person with a life-force that will project
out to everyone you meet. Good health
is your God given right. We have a lot to
look forward to. It would be great if you
could spend your life creating
experiences in a healthy state of mind
and body. Here is your beginning; a
healthy liver and body are waiting for
you. Let's get started.

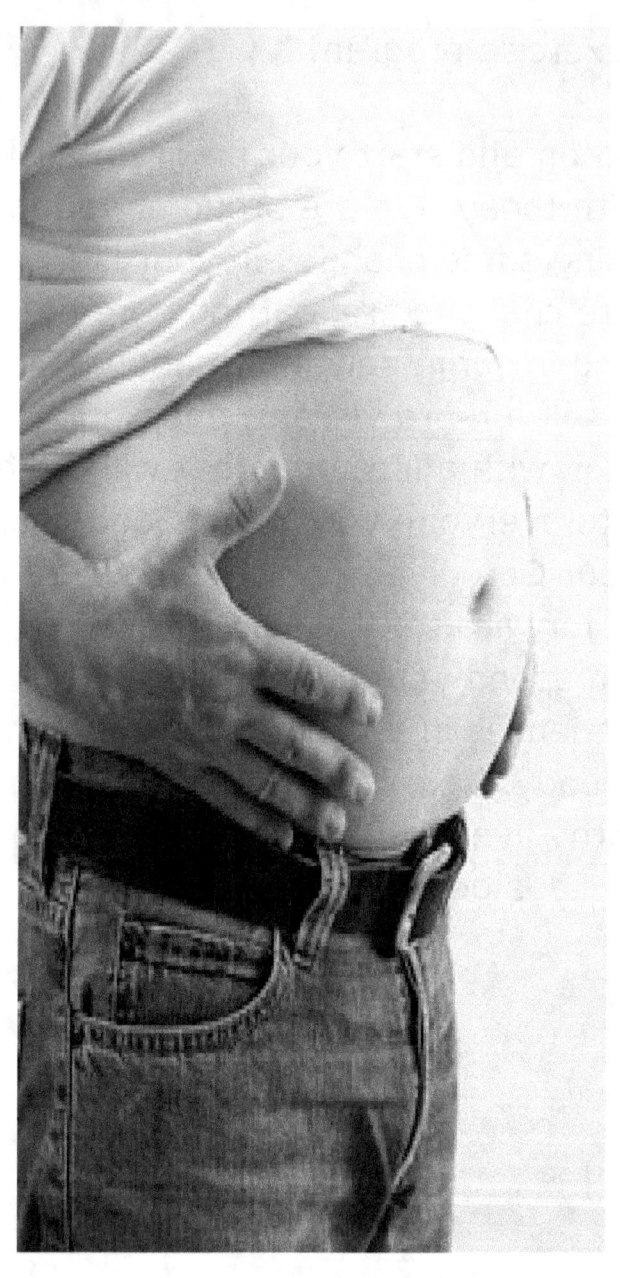

Energy

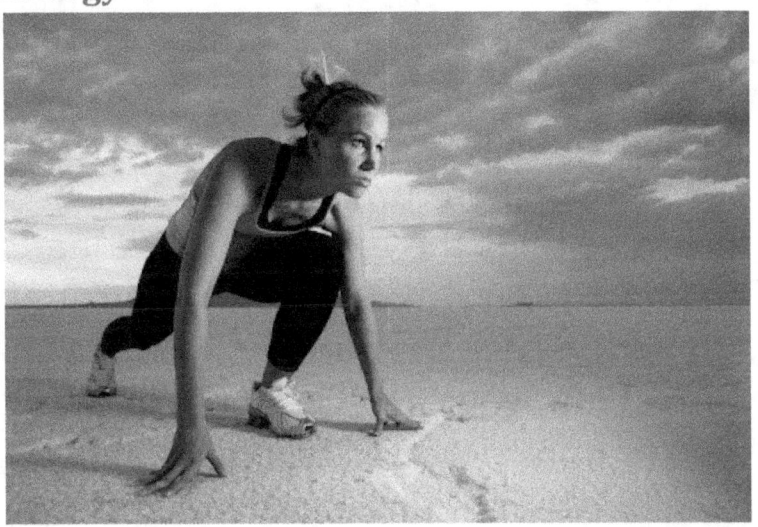

What is energy?

It is often understood as the ability a physical system has to do work on other physical systems. Since work is defined as a force acting through a distance (a length of space), energy is always equivalent to the ability to exert pulls or pushes against the basic forces of nature, along a path of a certain length.

The Wikipedia definition above simply means one's ability to use their body to accomplish a task. We all want more energy. Whether you do physical labor or white collar work, energy plays a role in our success or failure. If we are not getting enough energy, we are slowly suffocating in our own bodies. Your liver maintains the balance of food in and energy out. Your liver; if unhealthy, will not process the nutrients you are putting into your body in the form of food or drink. We will talk more about toxicity later but understand that toxins over run an unhealthy liver. Many of the ailments we face can be traced back to a toxic state.

Poor liver function means less energy to perform basic tasks. Why do so many people need the 2pm coffee to get through the rest of the day? Energy. Once your liver begins to clean itself; you will notice you have more energy and focus to get more things done. A healthy liver means no more yo-yo dieting; which is what we will be discussing in our next section. Get ready to finally keep those pounds off that you work so hard to lose.

Fat Just Keeps Coming Back!

Are you familiar with the phrase yo-yo dieting? This is an unhealthy cycle of losing weight and eventually putting it back on. You lose that 30 pounds and get all of those compliments. Fast forward 1 year. The 30 ponds are back and they didn't want to come back alone. They brought 10 more friends for a net gain of 40 pounds. Does this sound familiar?

Cirrhosis of the liver

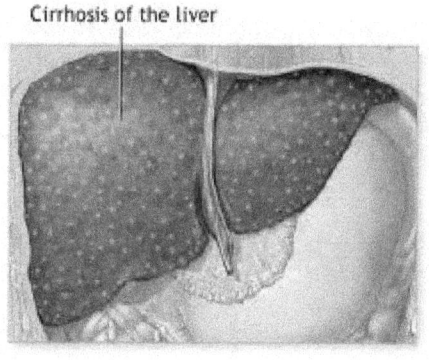

© ADAM, Inc.

Yo-yo diet syndrome is directly related to poor liver function. Poor liver function does not metabolize fat properly so you end up back where you started no matter how much time and hard work you put in. The only way you will have permanent weight loss will be through a clean, efficient running liver. Yes, your liver function can make you fat. Most people will never make this connection. They will, unfortunately, spend their time and resources trying to reach a goal that is both non-attainable and sustainable. We will provide you access to an eye opening video that will help you understand why poor liver function will keep you fat.

In the next section, we will talk about a few functions the liver performs.

Liver function

The liver performs over 500 different functions. Some of the important functions include:

- Assimilating and storing fat-soluble vitamins

- Creating bile
- Filtering blood
- Metabolizing fats, proteins, and carbohydrates
- Metabolizing hormones, internally-produced wastes, and foreign chemicals
- Producing urea (a primary waste product, flushed from the body in urine)
- Purifying and clearing waste products, toxins, and drugs
- Regulating and secreting substances important to maintaining body functions and health
- Storing important nutrients (such as glycogen glucose), vitamins, and minerals
- Synthesizing blood proteins

It is not important that you understand how all of this fits together. Just know that this super organ never stops working. The good news is that even if you have damaged your liver; there is a great chance that it will repair itself. Proper nutrition is the key to keeping your liver in shape. We will spend some time in the next section discussing how nutrition will impact your life.

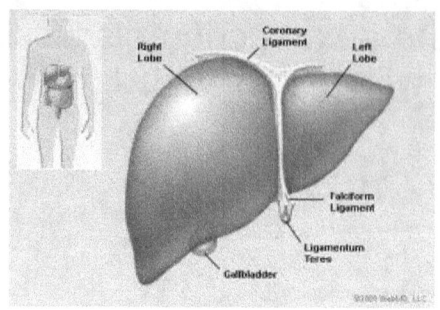

Foods That Feed the Liver

List of Foods that Cleanse the Liver

The only way to clean your liver is through nutrition. There are certain foods that can help restore your liver to a healthy state. Below is a list that will be a good starting point. Here is what we suggest to get your liver cleansed. Number one, find a good liver cleaning supplement and use it as directed. Number two, take 2 liver and gall bladder cleanses a year. Finally, eat the food listed below in abundance. You will begin to feel better, lose weight and feel more energetic. More importantly, your weight will begin to stabilize.

Garlic

1. Garlic

It doesn't take much for this white bulb to produce healthy results for the liver. The allicin and selenium are two fighters that aid in cleansing the liver of toxins. If you can handle it, try eating 1 clove of raw garlic 3 times a week. Watch the results!

Grapefruit

2. Grapefruit

High in both vitamin C and antioxidants, grapefruit intensifies the natural cleansing processes of the liver. Try drinking a small glass of freshly-squeezed grapefruit juice 4 times a week to help boost production of liver detoxification enzymes that help flush out carcinogens and other toxins.

Beets

3. Beets and Carrots

Both extremely high in plant-flavonoids and beta-carotene, eating both beets and carrots can help stimulate and improve overall liver function.

Green Tea

4. Green Tea

They are still documenting the benefits of this anti-oxidant laden beverage. Try switching to green tea. It tastes great and is kind to your liver.

Leafy Greens

5. Leafy Green Vegetables

Liver cleansing should always start with green leafy vegetables. Try going the raw route first although cooked and juiced can be healthy as well. Dense with energy giving plant chlorophylls, greens literally vacuum unhealthy toxins from the blood stream. One of the strongest properties of greens are their ability to neutralize heavy metals, pesticides and chemicals from the bloodstream aiding the liver.

Include leafy greens such as broccoli, bitter gourd, mustard greens and chicory into your eating arsenal. Other healthy greens include spinach, dandelion and chicory. Make a habit to add a green from the list to one meal every day. The more greens you eat; especially raw, the more bile is created to remove toxins from your blood. Remember, bile is your friend.

Avocado

6. Avocados

Glutathione is the main ingredient we get from avocados. Glutathione is another aid in cleaning toxins. The more you eat, the healthier your liver will become.

Apple

7. Apples

Pectin is the key here. The fiber from the apple helps clean the digestive tract. This allows the liver to work more efficiently. Don't kid yourself; an apple a day will prolong your life in many ways.

Olive Oil

8. Olive Oil

The big three; organic olive, hemp and flax-seed help the live when used in moderation. Cold-pressed is important. These oils aid the body by promoting a lipid base that engulfs harmful toxins in the body. This process takes some of the work off the liver in terms of the toxic taxing that many of us suffer from.

Whole Grains

9. Whole Grains

Grains, such as brown rice, are rich in B-complex vitamins, nutrients known to improve fat metabolism, liver function and liver decongestion. Do not eat foods with white flour, your liver will be better maintained with whole wheat alternatives.

Broccoli

10. Cruciferous Vegetables

What better way to increase enzyme production in the liver than eating cauliflower and broccoli. Glucosinolate is what we are getting here. Carcinogens are flushed out of the body with these enzymes. Smokers, while you are in the process of quitting; eat these two super foods.

Lemons and Limes

11. Lemons & Limes

These citrus fruits contain very high amounts of the vitamin C, which aids the body in synthesizing toxic material into substance that can be absorbed by water. Drinking freshly-squeezed lemon or lime juice in the morning helps stimulate the liver.

12. Walnuts

Walnuts

Holding high amount of the amino acid arginine, walnuts aid the liver in detoxifying ammonia. Walnuts are also high in glutathione and omega-3 fatty acids which support normal liver cleansing actions. Make sure you chew the nuts well (until they are liquefied) before swallowing.

Cabbage

13. Cabbage

Much like broccoli and cauliflower, eating cabbage helps stimulate the activation of two crucial liver detoxifying enzymes that help flush out toxins. Try eating more kimchi, coleslaw, cabbage soup and sauerkraut.

Turmeric Powder

14. Turmeric

The liver's favorite spice. Try adding some of this detoxifying goodness into your next lentil stew or veggie dish for an instant liver pick-me-up. Turmeric helps boost liver detox, by assisting enzymes that actively flush out known dietary carcinogens.

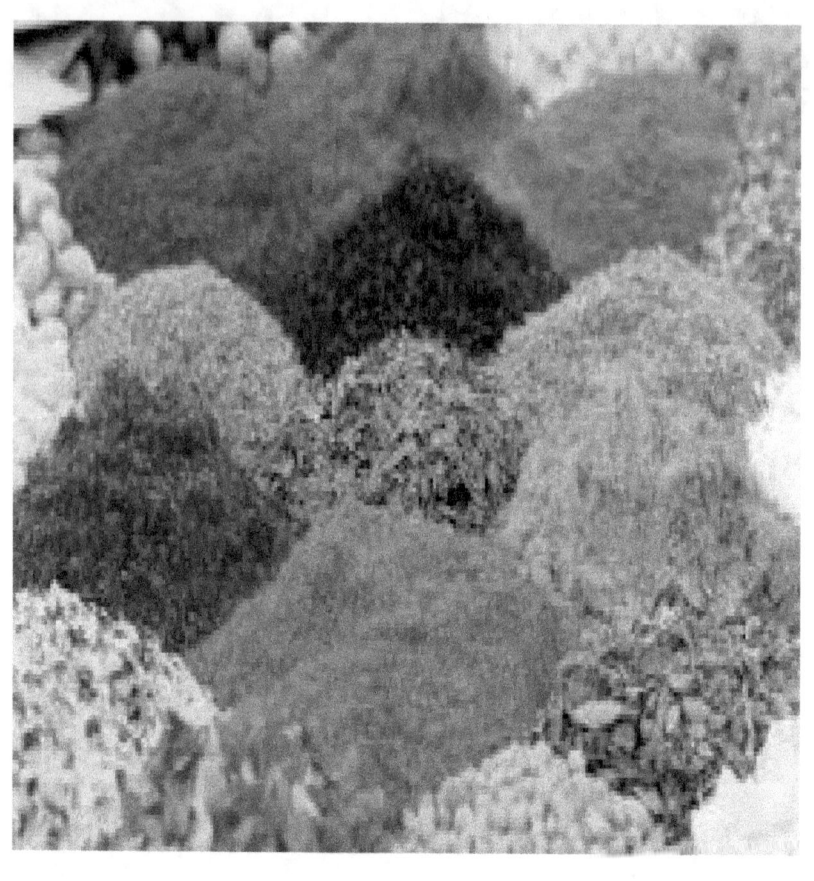

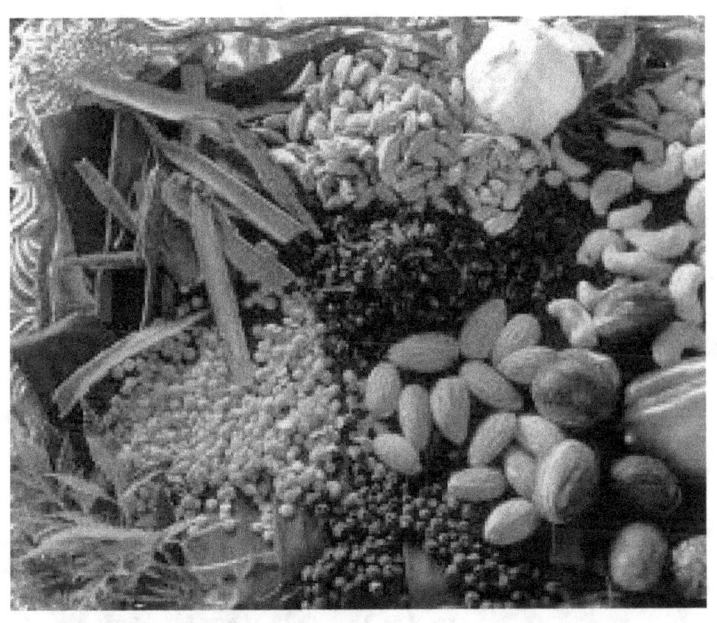

Foods That Hurt the Liver

Protein from animal sources provides vital nutrients and amino acids that the body needs. These foods are fine to eat if you have a healthy liver. When the liver is healthy, protein also helps the body repair tissue and prevents fat from accumulating in the cells. When the liver is damaged, it is unable to metabolize the protein sufficiently. This will cause an increase of toxins which are not broken down in normal liver process. Therefore; you must watch the amount of animal protein your body is talking in. You must actually limit animal protein until your liver is able to function properly. Animal source protein must be restricted in the diet to reduce the chance of toxic waste buildup due to poor liver processing. What are your healthy alternatives? Beans, nuts and wheat based products can provide the amino similar to what meat provide.

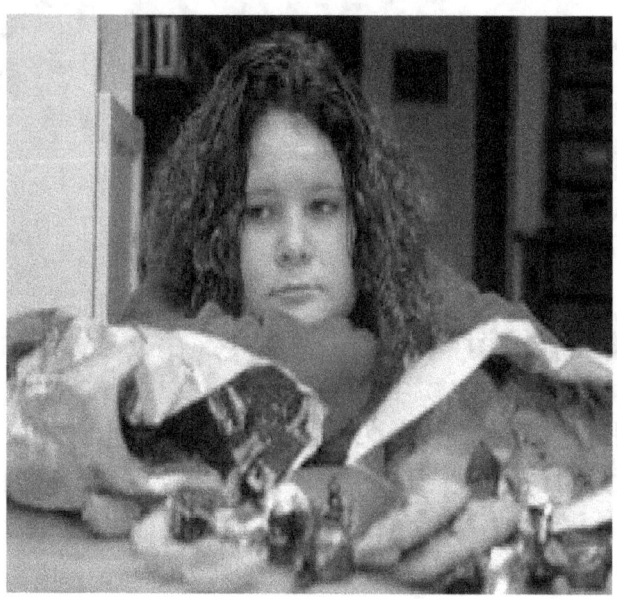

A damaged liver cannot process sodium efficiently. Do yourself a favor and avoid canned foods. These sodium rich products will cause abdominal swelling along with fluid retention. Fluid retention is a known precursor to hypertension! Use garlic, licorice and other spices in place of salt and sugar. These natural spices provide a boost to liver function. If you have salt and sugar cravings; try fresh fruit like strawberries or oranges. They provide a natural sweeteners and fiber which the body needs.

Do you have a beer-belly? That is your liver crying out for relief. You need to avoid alcohol for a period of time if you want to repair your liver. In fact, scientific evidence has proven that abstinence from alcohol; can result in total liver regeneration. Yes, you can give yourself a second chance if you exercise discipline for a period of time. Chronic alcohol consumption is surely a short trip to permanent liver damage and early death. Avoid drinking beer, wine or champagne as well as any form of liquor. Take note that some over-the-counter pain medications also contain alcohol, such as cough syrup.

Exercise for Liver Health

Exercise is good for your overall health. Make sure you seek out the advice of a health care professional before you begin any new physically exerting program.

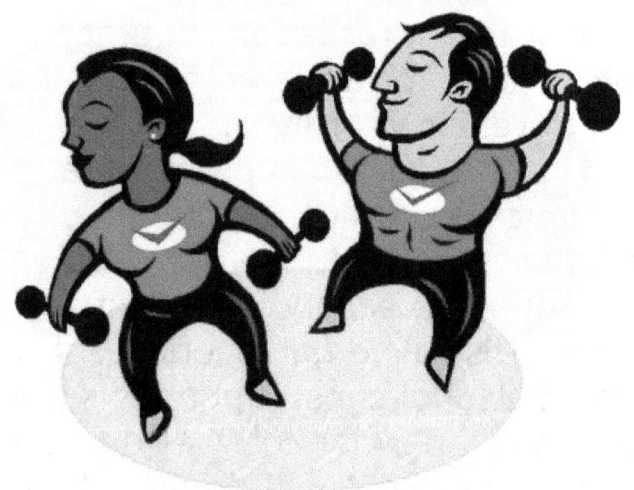

At minimum, you need to oxygenate your body. This can be done by walking. Walking on a treadmill at 3.5 mph is a good start. I would also recommend a 3.5 incline. Easy to remember; 3.5 and 3.5. That should be done 3 times a week minimum.

Here is something that is important to understand. Building muscle should be a goal that you and everyone strive for in your life. You should get involved in resistance training because it will strengthen your inner organs; especially the liver. Here is the formula to give you the quickest results in a short period of time.

The three large muscle groups you should focus on are the legs, chest and abdominal areas. If you focus on strengthening those 3 areas, you will be in great shape.

If you have access to a sauna, use it. Sweating toxins out of your body takes some of the load off of your liver. Infrared is best, dry heat second and finally steam. The first two options are the best.

Make a habit of doing something physical at least 3 times a week. Most health advocates recommend 4 days. The more time you can put into your physical well-being, the more return in terms of years will be achieved. Get off on the couch, put some motivating music in that MP3 player, and get it done.

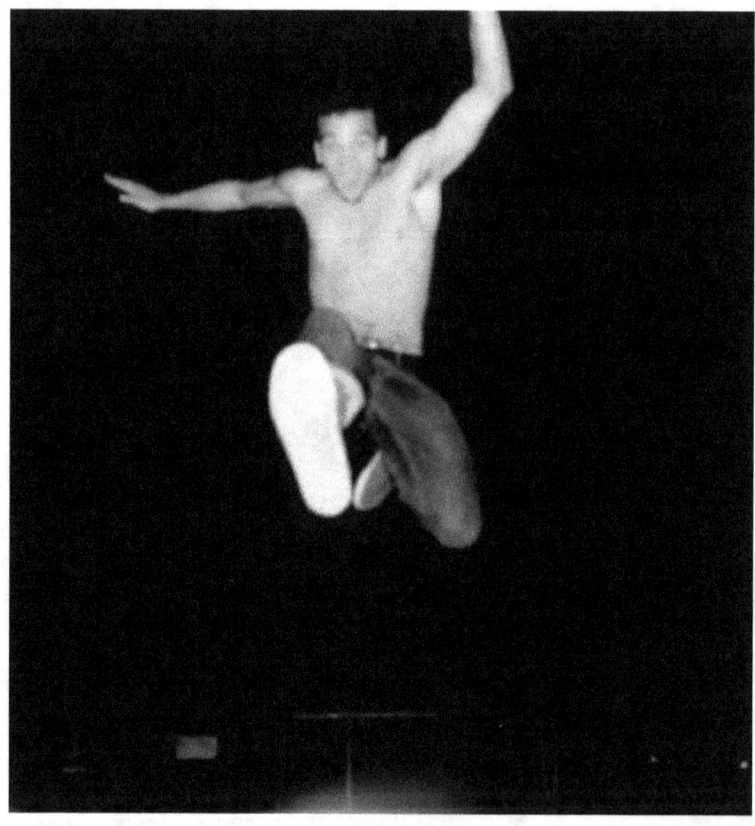

Conclusion

You now have some information to change your health. Act on it now. Obesity and other weight related ailments have become a public health crisis worldwide. We are getting fatter and sicker each year globally. You have to go to the mountains of Pakistan and other remote pockets to find declining numbers of obesity related illnesses.

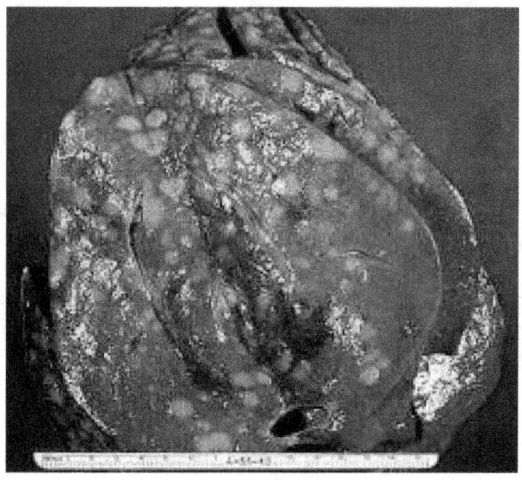

Make a commitment to yourself to not become a statistic. Making a few lifestyle changes and doing some occasional internal cleaning is all it takes. Junk food is not going to help you reach your goals. We are not suggesting you give up junk food altogether. An occasional snack is actually good for you. If you constantly crave junk, you will never have good health because you will eventually give in. Balance is the key. Put some balance and discipline in your life and you will win.

Your liver health is your lifeline. Your quality of life is tied to how you clean the toxic substances out of your body. Clean the filter and you will stay younger. Start exercising and stay younger. Eat more organic fruits and vegetables and stay younger. Give 3 compliments a day to 3 people and stay younger.

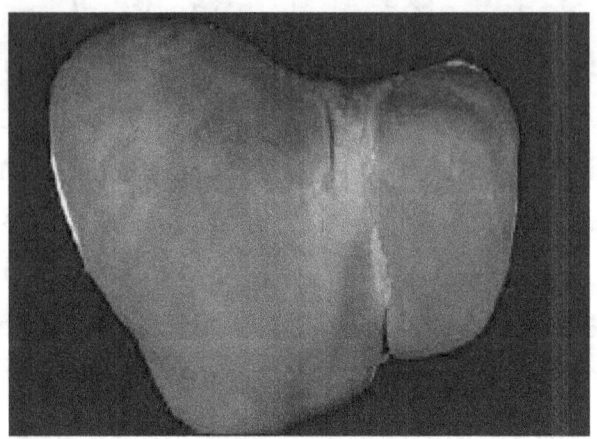

Take care of your liver and it will take care of you. The following resources are designed to help you in your journey.

Resources

Liver Cleanse –
www.nbiznow.com/healthy-liver

Fat Loss Factor – watch this video to see how the liver can keep you fat. This is a great solution.

www.nbiznow.com/fat-loss

Raw Food Diet – to get a great understanding of eating raw/live foods.

www.nbiznow.com/rawfood-diet

Free Downloads:

1. Ab Workouts http://nbiznow.com/Ab_Workouts-bonus.pdf
2. Beginners Yoga http://nbiznow.com/yoga-bonus.pdf

3. Total Fitness
   http://nbiznow.com/fitnessbook.pdf